Copyright © 2020 by Dr. Adel Tundey

All rights reserved. No part of this publication may be reproduced, distributed, or transmitted in any form or by any means, including photocopying, recording, or other electronic or mechanical methods, without the prior written permission of the publisher, except in the case of brief quotations embodied in critical reviews and certain other noncommercial uses permitted by copyright law.

Table of Contents

INTRODUCTION 4

CANCER 6

    Types of Cancer 8

    Symptoms Of Cancer 37

    Causes Of Cancer 39

    Diagnosis of Cancer 49

BEETROOT 51

    Nutrition 51

    Benefits 53

CARROT 57

    Nutrition 57

    Vitamins and Minerals 60

    Other Plant Compounds 60

    Health benefits of carrots 62

APPLE 64

    Nutrition 64

    Benefits 66

        Neurological health and dementia 67

    Dietary tips and recipes 71

LEMON 73

    Nutrition 73

    Benefits 74

- Vitamin C 80
- **BEETROOT, CARROT, APPLE AND LEMON FOR CANCER** 82
  - How Does The Miracle Drink Fight Cancer? 84
    - How To Make Miracle Drink For Cancer 84
  - Recipe of ABC Miracle Drink 85
    - Ingredients you'll need: 85
    - How to Prepare: 85
    - When to Drink it: 86
  - Dosage 86
- **CONCLUSION** 87

INTRODUCTION

A magic potion that has gained worldwide fame for its amazing effects on health. For the first time began to be used in the traditional Chinese medicine in the treatment of lung cancer and various other diseases. He came to the conclusion that malignant tumor cells can survive only with the help of strong meat. He has created the therapy for a period of 42 days during which the patient may be in your body to enter only teas and special vegetable juice, whose main ingredient are beetroot, carrot, apple and lemon. With the help of this method of cure over 45,000 people with cancer and other terminal illnesses.

This simple drink miraculous properties owes to the presence of two modest vegetables and one type of fruit. Their medicinal properties, many of you are already well known.

Beetroot is rich in vitamins A, C and B and iron, copper, magnesium and potassium. It is known for its beneficial effects on the heart, blood vessels, liver and entire digestive system, and as a natural substance that protects against cancer.

The carrot is famous for vitamins A, B, C, E and K. It contains the minerals calcium, magnesium, potassium and selenium. It is natural asset that preserves vision, reduces the risk of stroke and has a strong anticancer effect.

Apple is rich in vitamins A, B complex, C, E and K, and the minerals zinc, magnesium, potassium, phosphorus, calcium, sodium and iron. Thanks to the high concentration of carbohydrates, especially fructose and glucose, Apple provides the body with energy and prevents fatigue. Due to the high content of vitamin C and antioxidants, apple has a strong immunostimulatory effect. It is very effective in fighting viruses, bacteria and free radicals, promotes weight loss and stimulates digestion.

Lemon are a popular fruit that people use in small quantities to add flavor to food. However, they rarely consume them alone due to their intense, sour taste.

Lemons give flavor to baked goods, sauces, salad dressings, marinades, drinks, and desserts, and they are also a good source of vitamin C.

CANCER

Cancer is a group of diseases involving abnormal cell growth with the potential to invade or spread to other parts of the body. These contrast with benign tumors, which do not spread. Possible signs and symptoms include a lump, abnormal bleeding, prolonged cough, unexplained weight loss, and a change in bowel movements. While these symptoms may indicate cancer, they can also have other causes. Over 100 types of cancers affect humans.

Tobacco use is the cause of about 22% of cancer deaths. Another 10% are due to obesity, poor diet, lack of physical activity or excessive drinking of alcohol. Other factors include certain infections, exposure to ionizing radiation and environmental pollutants. In the developing world, 15% of cancers are due to infections such as Helicobacter pylori, hepatitis B, hepatitis C, human papillomavirus infection, Epstein–Barr virus and human immunodeficiency virus (HIV). These factors act, at least partly, by changing the genes of a cell. Typically, many genetic changes are required before cancer develops. Approximately 5–10% of cancers are due to inherited genetic defects from a person's parents. Cancer can be detected by certain signs and symptoms or screening tests. It is then typically further investigated by medical imaging and confirmed by biopsy.

Many cancers can be prevented by not smoking, maintaining a healthy weight, not drinking too much alcohol, eating plenty of vegetables, fruits and whole grains, vaccination against certain infectious diseases, not eating too much processed and red meat and avoiding too much sunlight exposure. Early detection through screening is useful for cervical and colorectal cancer. The benefits of screening in breast cancer are controversial. Cancer is often treated with some combination of radiation therapy, surgery, chemotherapy and targeted therapy. Pain and symptom management are an important part of care. Palliative care is particularly important in people with advanced disease. The chance of survival depends on the type of cancer and extent of disease at the start of treatment. In children under 15 at diagnosis, the five-year survival rate in the developed world is on average 80%. For cancer in the United States, the average five-year survival rate is 66%.

In 2015, about 90.5 million people had cancer. About 14.1 million new cases occur a year (not including skin cancer other than melanoma). It caused about 8.8 million deaths (15.7% of deaths). The most common types of cancer in males are lung cancer, prostate cancer, colorectal cancer and stomach cancer.[19] In females, the most common types are breast cancer, colorectal cancer, lung cancer and cervical cancer.[11] If skin cancer other than melanoma were included in total new cancer cases each year, it would account for around 40% of cases. In children, acute lymphoblastic leukemia and brain tumors are most common, except in Africa where non-Hodgkin lymphoma occurs more often. In 2012, about 165,000 children under 15 years of age were diagnosed with cancer. The risk of cancer increases significantly with age, and many cancers occur more commonly in developed countries. Rates are increasing as more people live to an old age and as lifestyle changes occur in the developing world. The financial costs of cancer were estimated at $1.16 trillion USD per year as of 2010.

Types of Cancer

Breast cancer

Cancer begins when healthy cells in the breast change and grow out of control, forming a mass or sheet of cells called a tumor. A tumor can be cancerous or benign. A cancerous tumor is malignant, meaning it can grow and spread to other parts of the body. A benign tumor means the tumor can grow but will not spread.

Breast cancer spreads when the cancer grows into other parts of the body or when breast cancer cells move to other parts of the body through the blood vessels and/or lymph vessels. This is called a metastasis.

This guide covers early-stage and locally advanced breast cancer, which includes stages I, II, and III. The stage of breast cancer describes where the cancer is located, how much the cancer has grown, and if or where it has spread.

Although breast cancer most commonly spreads to nearby lymph nodes, it can also spread further through the body to areas such as the bones, lungs, liver, and brain. This is called metastatic or stage IV breast cancer. Learn more about metastatic breast cancer in a separate section on this website.

If breast cancer comes back after initial treatment, it can recur locally, meaning in the breast and/or regional lymph nodes. The regional lymph nodes are those nearby the breast, such as the lymph nodes under the arm. It can also recur elsewhere in the body, called a distant recurrence or metastatic recurrence.

Types of breast cancer

Breast cancer can be invasive or noninvasive. Invasive breast cancer is cancer that spreads into surrounding tissues. Noninvasive breast cancer does not go beyond the milk ducts or lobules in the breast. Most breast cancers start in the ducts or lobes and are called ductal carcinoma or lobular carcinoma:

- Ductal carcinoma. These cancers start in the cells lining the milk ducts and make up the majority of breast cancers.
    - Ductal carcinoma in situ (DCIS). This is cancer that is located only in the duct.
    - Invasive or infiltrating ductal carcinoma. This is cancer that has spread outside of the duct.
- Invasive lobular carcinoma. This is cancer that starts in the lobules.

Less common types of breast cancer include:

- Medullary
- Mucinous
- Tubular
- Metaplastic
- Papillary

- Inflammatory breast cancer is a faster-growing type of cancer that accounts for about 1% to 5% of all breast cancers.
- Paget's disease is a type of cancer that begins in the ducts of the nipple. Although it is usually in situ, it can also be an invasive cancer.

Bladder Cancer

Bladder cancer begins when healthy cells in the bladder lining—most commonly urothelial cells—change and grow out of control, forming a mass called a tumor. Urothelial cells also line the renal pelvis and ureters. Cancer that develops in the renal pelvis and ureters is also considered a type of bladder cancer and is often called upper tract bladder cancer. It is treated in the same way as bladder cancer and is described in this guide. A tumor can be cancerous or benign. A cancerous tumor is malignant, meaning it can grow and spread to other parts of the body. A benign tumor means the tumor can grow but will not spread. Benign bladder tumors are rare.

Types of bladder cancer

The type of bladder cancer depends on how the tumor's cells look under the microscope. The 3 main types of bladder cancer are:

- Urothelial carcinoma. Urothelial carcinoma (or UCC) accounts for about 90% of all bladder cancers. It also accounts for 10% to 15% of kidney cancers diagnosed in adults. It begins in the urothelial cells found in the urinary tract. Urothelial carcinoma is sometimes also called transitional cell carcinoma or TCC.
- Squamous cell carcinoma. Squamous cells develop in the bladder lining in response to irritation and inflammation. Over time, these cells may become cancerous. Squamous cell carcinoma accounts for about 4% of all bladder cancers.
- Adenocarcinoma. This type accounts for about 2% of all bladder cancers and develops from glandular cells.

There are other, less common types of bladder cancer, including sarcoma of the bladder and small cell bladder cancer. Sarcomas of the bladder often begin in the fat or muscle layers of the bladder. Small cell bladder cancer is a rare type of bladder cancer that is likely to spread to other parts of the body.

Other ways of describing bladder cancer

In addition to its cell type, bladder cancer may be described as noninvasive, non-muscle-invasive, or muscle-invasive.

- Noninvasive. Noninvasive bladder cancer includes noninvasive papillary carcinoma and carcinoma in situ (CIS). Noninvasive papillary carcinoma is a growth found on a small section of tissue that is easily removed. This is called stage 0a. CIS is cancer that is found only on or near the surface of the bladder, which is called stage 0is.
- Non-muscle-invasive. Non-muscle-invasive bladder cancer typically has only grown into the lamina propria and not into muscle, also called stage I. Non-muscle-invasive cancer may also be called superficial cancer, although this term is being used less often because it may incorrectly suggest that this type of cancer is not serious.
- Muscle-invasive. Muscle-invasive bladder cancer has grown into the bladder's wall muscle and sometimes into the fatty layers or surrounding tissue outside the bladder.

It is important to note that non-muscle-invasive bladder cancer has the possibility of spreading into the bladder muscle or to other parts of the body. Additionally, all cell types of bladder cancer can spread beyond the bladder to other areas of the body through a process known as metastasis.

If a bladder tumor has spread into the surrounding organs, such as the uterus and vagina in women, the prostate in men, and/or nearby muscles, it is called locally advanced disease. Bladder cancer also often spreads to the lymph nodes in the pelvis. If it has spread into the liver, bones, lungs, lymph nodes outside the pelvis, or other parts of the body, the cancer is called metastatic disease.

Colorectal Cancer

Colorectal cancer begins when healthy cells in the lining of the colon or rectum change and grow out of control, forming a mass called a tumor. A tumor can be cancerous or benign. A cancerous tumor is malignant, meaning it can grow and spread to other parts of the body. A benign tumor means the tumor can grow but will not spread. These changes usually take years to develop. Both genetic and environmental factors can cause the changes. However, when a person has an uncommon inherited syndrome, changes can occur in months or years.

Anatomy of the colon and rectum

The colon and rectum make up the large intestine, which plays an important role in the body's ability to process waste. The colon makes up the first 5 to 6 feet of the large intestine, and the rectum makes up the last 6 inches, ending at the anus.

The colon and rectum have 5 sections. The ascending colon is the portion that extends from a pouch called the cecum. The cecum is the beginning of the large intestine into which the small intestine empties; it's on the right side of the abdomen. The transverse colon crosses the top of the abdomen. The descending colon takes waste down the left side. Finally, the sigmoid colon at the bottom takes waste a few more inches, down to the rectum. Waste leaves the body through the anus.

colorectal polyps

Colorectal cancer most often begins as a polyp, a noncancerous growth that may develop on the inner wall of the colon or rectum as people get older. If not treated or removed, a polyp can become a potentially life-threatening cancer. Finding and removing precancerous polyps can prevent colorectal cancer.

There are several forms of polyps. Adenomatous polyps, or adenomas, are growths that may become cancerous. They can be found with a colonoscopy. Polyps are most easily found during a colonoscopy because they usually bulge into the colon, forming a mound on the wall of the colon that can be found by the doctor.

About 10% of colon polyps are flat and hard to find with a colonoscopy unless a dye is used to highlight them. These flat polyps have a high risk of becoming cancerous, regardless of their size.

Hyperplastic polyps may also develop in the colon and rectum. They are not considered precancerous.

Types of colorectal cancer

Colorectal cancer can begin in either the colon or the rectum. Cancer that begins in the colon is called colon cancer. Cancer that begins in the rectum is called rectal cancer.

Most colon and rectal cancers are a type of tumor called adenocarcinoma, which is cancer of the cells that line the inside tissue of the colon and rectum. This section specifically covers adenocarcinoma. Other types of cancer that occur far less often but can begin in the colon or rectum include neuroendocrine tumor of the gastrointestinal tract, gastrointestinal stromal tumor (GIST), small cell carcinoma, and lymphoma.

kidney cancer

Kidney cancer begins when healthy cells in 1 or both kidneys change and grow out of control, forming a mass called a renal cortical tumor. A tumor can be malignant, indolent, or benign. A malignant tumor is cancerous, meaning it can grow and spread to other parts of the body. An indolent tumor is also cancerous, but this type of tumor rarely spreads to other parts of the body. A benign tumor means the tumor can grow but will not spread.

Types of kidney cancer

There are several types of kidney cancer:

- Renal cell carcinoma. Renal cell carcinoma is the most common type of adult kidney cancer, making up about 85% of diagnoses. This type of cancer develops in the proximal renal tubules that make up the kidney's filtration system. There are thousands of these tiny filtration units in each kidney. The treatment options for renal cell carcinoma are discussed later in this guide.
- Urothelial carcinoma. This is also called transitional cell carcinoma. It accounts for 10% to 15% of the kidney cancers diagnosed in adults. Urothelial carcinoma begins in the area of the kidney where urine collects before moving to the bladder, called the renal pelvis. This type of kidney cancer is treated like bladder cancer because both types of cancer start in the same cells.

- Sarcoma. Sarcoma of the kidney is rare. This type of cancer develops in the soft tissue of the kidney; the thin layer of connective tissue surrounding the kidney, called the capsule; or surrounding fat. Sarcoma of the kidney is usually treated with surgery. However, sarcoma commonly comes back in the kidney area or spreads to other parts of the body. More surgery or chemotherapy may be recommended after the first surgery.
- Wilms tumor. Wilms tumor is most common in children and is treated differently from kidney cancer in adults. This type of tumor is more likely to be successfully treated with radiation therapy and chemotherapy than the other types of kidney cancer when combined with surgery. This has resulted in a different approach to treatment.
- Lymphoma. Lymphoma can enlarge both kidneys and is associated with enlarged lymph nodes, called lymphadenopathy, in other parts of the body, including the neck, chest, and abdominal cavity. In rare cases, kidney lymphoma can appear as a lone tumor mass in the kidney and may include enlarged regional lymph nodes. If lymphoma is a possibility, your doctor may perform a biopsy (see Diagnosis) and recommend chemotherapy instead of surgery.

Types of kidney cancer cells

Knowing which type of cell makes up a kidney tumor helps doctors plan treatment. Pathologists have identified as many as 20 different types of kidney cancer cells. A pathologist is a doctor who specializes in interpreting laboratory tests and evaluating cells, tissues, and organs to diagnose disease. Computed tomography (CT) scans or magnetic resonance imaging (MRI) cannot always distinguish between benign, indolent, or malignant renal cortical tumors before surgery.

The most common types of kidney cancer cells are listed below.

- Clear cell. About 70% of kidney cancers are made up of clear cells. Clear cells range from slow growing (grade 1) to fast growing (grade 4). Immunotherapy and targeted therapy are particularly effective at treating clear cell kidney cancer.
- Papillary. Papillary kidney cancer develops in 10% to 15% of patients. It is divided into 2 different subtypes, called type 1 and type 2. Papillary kidney cancer is currently treated in the same way as clear cell kidney cancer. However, many doctors recommend treatment through a clinical trial because treatment with targeted therapy is

often not as successful for people with papillary kidney cancer as it is for people with clear cell kidney cancer.
- Sarcomatoid features. Each of the tumor subtypes of clear cell, chromophobe, and papillary in kidney cancer can show highly disorganized features under the microscope. These are often described by pathologists as "sarcomatoid." This is not a distinct tumor subtype, but when these features are seen, doctors are aware that this is a very aggressive form of kidney cancer.
- Medullary/collecting duct. This is a rare and highly aggressive cancer that is closely related to transitional cell carcinoma (see above) but is still considered a renal cortical tumor. It is more common in black people and is highly associated with having the sickle cell trait. Sickle cell trait means that a person has inherited the sickle cell gene from a parent. Collecting duct is more likely to occur in people between the ages of 20 and 30. Despite combinations of systemic chemotherapy and surgery, this form of kidney cancer has lower long-term survival rates.
- Chromophobe. Chromophobe is another uncommon cancer that is different from the other types. It may form indolent tumors.

- Oncocytoma. This is a slow-growing type of kidney cancer that rarely, if ever, spreads.
- Angiomyolipoma. Angiomyolipoma is a benign tumor that has a unique appearance on a CT (or CAT) scan and when viewed under a microscope. Usually, it is less likely to grow and spread. It is generally best treated with surgery or, if it is small, active surveillance. An aggressive form of angiomyolipoma, called epithelioid, can in rare instances spread to nearby lymph nodes or organs such as the liver.

Non-Small Cell Lung Cancer

There are 2 main classifications of lung cancer: small cell lung cancer and non-small cell lung cancer (NSCLC). These 2 types are treated differently. This guide contains information about NSCLC.

NSCLC begins when healthy cells in the lung change and grow out of control, forming a mass called a tumor, a lesion, or a nodule. A lung tumor can begin anywhere in the lung. A tumor can be cancerous or benign. Once a cancerous lung tumor grows, it may shed cancer cells. These cells can be carried away in blood or float away in the fluid, called lymph, that surrounds lung tissue. Lymph flows through tubes called lymphatic vessels that drain into collecting stations called lymph nodes. Lymph nodes are the tiny, bean-shaped organs that help fight infection. They are located in the lungs, the center of the chest, and elsewhere in the body. The natural flow of lymph out of the lungs is toward the center of the chest, which explains why lung cancer often spreads there first. When a cancer cell moves into a lymph node or to a distant part of the body through the bloodstream, it is called metastasis.

Types of NSCLC

NSCLC begins in the epithelial cells. NSCLC may also be described based on the type of epithelial cell where the cancer starts:

- Adenocarcinoma starts in cells that produce mucus.
- Squamous cell carcinoma begins in the cells that line the airways.
- Large cell carcinoma begins in cells other than the 2 types described above.

It is important for doctors to distinguish between lung cancer that begins in the squamous cells from lung cancer that begins in other cells. This information is used to determine treatment options.

Normal lung tissue

Lung - adenocarcinoma

Lung - squamous cell carcinoma.

non-Hodgkin lymphoma

Lymphoma is a cancer of the lymphatic system. Lymphoma begins when healthy B cells, T cells, or NK cells in the lymphatic system change and grow out of control, which may form a tumor. Hodgkin lymphoma is a specific type of lymphoma. Non-Hodgkin lymphoma (NHL) is a term that refers to a group of cancers of the lymphatic system. These cancers can have different symptoms and signs, findings on a physical examination, and treatments.

Because lymphatic tissue is found in most parts of the body, NHL can start almost anywhere and can spread, or metastasize, to almost any organ. It often begins in the lymph nodes, liver, spleen, or bone marrow. However, it can also involve the stomach, intestines, skin, thyroid gland, brain, or any other part of the body.

It is very important to know which type and subtype of lymphoma has been diagnosed. That information can help the doctor figure out the best treatment, as well as a patient's prognosis, which is the chance of recovery.

Melanoma

The deepest layer of the epidermis, located just above the dermis, contains cells called melanocytes. Melanocytes produce the skin's pigment or color. Melanoma begins when healthy melanocytes change and grow out of control, forming a cancerous tumor. A cancerous tumor is malignant, meaning it can grow and spread to other parts of the body. Sometimes, melanoma develops from a normal mole a person already has on their skin. When this happens, the mole will undergo changes that usually can be seen, such as changes in shape, size, color, or the border of the mole.

Melanoma can develop anywhere on the body, including the head and neck, the skin under the fingernails, the genitals, and even the soles of the feet or palms of the hands. Melanoma may not be colored like a mole. It may have no color or be slightly red, which is called amelanotic melanoma.

When found early, melanoma can often be cured with surgery. However, melanoma is 1 of the most serious forms of skin cancer. It can grow deep into the skin, called invasive melanoma. It can also invade lymph nodes and blood vessels and spread to distant parts of the body, called metastatic melanoma.

This section focuses on cutaneous melanoma, which is melanoma that first develops in the skin. Melanoma can also develop in the mucous membranes that line the mouth, the gastrointestinal tract, a woman's vagina, and other locations around the body. Melanoma may also develop in the eye. Learn more about melanoma diagnosed in other parts of the body in these separate sections:

- Melanoma of the eye
- Melanoma of the anus
- Melanoma of the vagina

Oral and Oropharyngeal Cancer

Cancer of the oral cavity and cancer of the oropharynx are 2 of the most common types of cancer that develop in the head and neck region, a grouping called head and neck cancer. The oral cavity and oropharynx, along with other parts of the head and neck, give us the ability to chew, swallow, breathe, and talk.

The oral cavity includes the:

- Lips
- Lining of the lips and cheeks, called the buccal mucosa
- Gingiva, which is the upper and lower gums

- Front two-thirds of the tongue
- Floor of the mouth under the tongue
- Hard palate, also called the roof of the mouth
- Retromolar trigone, which is the small area behind the wisdom teeth

The oropharynx begins where the oral cavity stops. It includes the:

- Soft palate at the back of the mouth
- Part of the throat behind the mouth
- Tonsils
- Base of the tongue

More than 90% of oral and oropharyngeal cancers are squamous cell carcinoma. This means that they begin in the flat, squamous cells found in the lining of the mouth and throat. The most common locations for cancer in the oral cavity are:

- Tongue
- Tonsils
- Oropharynx
- Gums
- Floor of the mouth

Although oral cancer and oropharyngeal cancer are commonly described using 1 phrase, it is important to identify exactly where the cancer began. This is because there are differences in treatment between the 2 locations.

The Pancreas

The pancreas is a pear-shaped gland located in the abdomen between the stomach and the spine. It is made up of 2 major components:

- The exocrine component is made up of ducts and small sacs called acini on the end of the ducts. This part of the pancreas makes specialized proteins called enzymes that are released into the small intestine to help the body digest and break down food, particularly fats.
- The endocrine component of the pancreas is made up of cells lumped together in different locations within this part of the pancreas, called islets of Langerhans. These cells make specific hormones, most importantly insulin. Insulin is the substance that helps control the amount of sugar in the blood. This portion of the pancreas also makes other hormones, such as glucagon, somatostatin, pancreatic polypeptide (PP), and vasoactive intestinal peptide (VIP).

Each of these hormones plays an important role in regulating the body's metabolism.

Types of pancreatic cancer

There are several types of pancreatic cancer, depending on whether the cancer began in the exocrine or endocrine component. Rarely, other types of cancer can begin in the pancreas, such as lymphoma and sarcoma.

- Exocrine tumors. These are the most common type of pancreatic cancer. And adenocarcinoma is the most common type of exocrine tumor. These tumors usually start in the ducts of the pancreas, called ductal adenocarcinoma. Much less commonly, if the tumor begins in the acini, it is called acinar adenocarcinoma.

  An increasingly common diagnosis is called intraductal papillary mucinous neoplasm (IPMN). An IPMN is a tumor that grows within the ducts of the pancreas and makes a thick fluid called mucin. IPMN is not cancerous when it begins but could become cancerous if not treated. Sometimes, an IPMN has already worsened and become a cancer by the time it is diagnosed.

Much rarer types of exocrine pancreatic tumors include: acinar cell carcinoma, adenosquamous carcinoma, colloid carcinoma, giant cell tumor, hepatoid carcinoma, mucinous cystic neoplasms, pancreatoblastoma, serous cystadenoma, signet ring cell carcinoma, solid and pseudopapillary tumors, squamous cell carcinoma, and undifferentiated carcinoma.

- Endocrine tumors. These are also called pancreatic neuroendocrine tumors (PNETs) or islet cell tumors. They are much less common than exocrine tumors, making up about 7% of pancreatic cancers. A pancreatic neuroendocrine tumor can be functioning or nonfunctioning. A functioning tumor makes hormones. A nonfunctioning tumor does not make hormones. A functioning neuroendocrine tumor is named based on the hormone the cells normally make. These include:
    - Insulinoma
    - Glucagonoma
    - Gastrinoma
    - Somatostatinoma
    - VIPomas
    - PPomas

Prostate Cancer

Cancer begins when healthy cells in the prostate change and grow out of control, forming a tumor. A tumor can be cancerous or benign. A cancerous tumor is malignant, meaning it can grow and spread to other parts of the body. A benign tumor means the tumor can grow but will not spread.

Prostate cancer is somewhat unusual when compared with other types of cancer. This is because many prostate tumors do not spread quickly to other parts of the body. Some prostate cancers grow very slowly and may not cause symptoms or problems for years or ever. Even when prostate cancer has spread to other parts of the body, it often can be managed for a long time, allowing men even with advanced prostate cancer to live with good health and quality of life for many years. However, if the cancer cannot be well controlled with existing treatments, it can cause symptoms like pain and fatigue and can sometimes lead to death. An important part of managing prostate cancer is monitoring it for growth over time, to determine whether it is growing slowly or quickly. Based on the pattern of growth, your doctor can decide the best available treatment options and when to give them.

The Thyroid

Thyroid cancer begins in the thyroid gland. This gland is located in the front of the neck just below the larynx, which is called the voice box. The thyroid gland is part of the endocrine system, which regulates hormones in the body. The thyroid gland absorbs iodine from the bloodstream to produce thyroid hormones, which regulate a person's metabolism.

A normal thyroid gland has 2 lobes, 1 on each side of the windpipe, joined by a narrow strip of tissue called the isthmus. A healthy thyroid gland is barely palpable, which means it is hard to find by touch. If a tumor develops in the thyroid, it is felt as a lump in the neck. A swollen or enlarged thyroid gland is called a goiter, which may be caused when a person does not get enough iodine. However, most Americans receive enough iodine from salt, and a goiter under these circumstances is caused by other reasons.

Thyroid Tumors

Thyroid cancer starts when healthy cells in the thyroid change and grow out of control, forming a mass called a tumor. The thyroid gland contains 2 types of cells:

- Follicular cells. These cells are responsible for the production of thyroid hormone. Thyroid hormone is needed to live. The hormone controls the basic metabolism of the body. It controls how quickly calories are burned. This can affect weight loss and weight gain, slow down or speed up the heartbeat, raise or lower body temperature, influence how quickly food moves through the digestive tract, control the way muscles contract, and control how quickly dying cells are replaced.
- C cells. These special cells of the thyroid make calcitonin, a hormone that participates in calcium metabolism.

A tumor can be cancerous or benign. A cancerous tumor is malignant, meaning it can grow and spread to other parts of the body. A benign tumor means the tumor can grow but will not spread. Thyroid tumors can also be called nodules, and about 90% of all thyroid nodules are benign.

Types of Thyroid Cancer

There are 5 main types of thyroid cancer:

- Papillary thyroid cancer. Papillary thyroid cancer develops from follicular cells and usually grow slowly. It is the most common type of thyroid cancer. It is usually found in 1 lobe. Only 10% to 20% of papillary thyroid cancer appears in both lobes. It is a differentiated thyroid cancer, meaning that the tumor looks similar to normal thyroid tissue under a microscope. Papillary thyroid cancer can often spread to lymph nodes.

- Follicular thyroid cancer. Follicular thyroid cancer also develops from follicular cells and usually grows slowly. Follicular thyroid cancer is also a differentiated thyroid cancer, but it is far less common than papillary thyroid cancer. Follicular thyroid cancer rarely spreads to lymph nodes.

Follicular thyroid cancer and papillary thyroid cancer are the most common differentiated thyroid cancers. They are very often curable, especially when found early and in people younger than 50. Together, follicular and papillary thyroid cancers make up about 95% of all thyroid cancer.

- Hurthle cell cancer. Hurthle cell cancer, also called Hurthle cell carcinoma, is cancer that is arises from a certain type of follicular cell. Hurthle cell cancers are much more likely to spread to lymph nodes than other follicular thyroid cancers.

- Medullary thyroid cancer (MTC). MTC develops in the C cells and is sometimes the result of a genetic syndrome called multiple endocrine neoplasia type 2 (MEN2). This tumor has very little, if any, similarity to normal thyroid tissue. MTC can often be controlled if it is diagnosed and treated before it spreads to other parts of the body. MTC accounts for about 3% of all thyroid cancers. About 25% of all MTC is familial. This means that family members of the patient will have a possibility of a similar diagnosis. The RET proto-oncogene test (see Risk Factors) can confirm if family members also have familial MTC (FMTC).
- Anaplastic thyroid cancer. This type is rare, accounting for about 1% of thyroid cancer. It is a fast-growing, poorly differentiated thyroid cancer that may start from differentiated thyroid cancer or a benign thyroid tumor. Anaplastic thyroid cancer can be subtyped into giant cell classifications. Because this type of thyroid cancer grows so quickly, it is more difficult to treat successfully.

Uterine Cancer

Uterine cancer is the most common cancer occurring in a woman's reproductive system. Uterine cancer begins when healthy cells in the uterus change and grow out of control, forming a mass called a tumor. A tumor can be cancerous or benign. A cancerous tumor is malignant, meaning it can grow and spread to other parts of the body. A benign tumor can grow but generally will not spread into other tissues.

Noncancerous conditions of the uterus include:

- Fibroids: Benign tumors in the muscle of the uterus
- Benign polyps: Abnormal growths in the lining of the uterus
- Endometriosis: A condition in which endometrial tissue, which usually lines the inside of the uterus, is found on the outside of the uterus or other organs.
- Endometrial hyperplasia: A condition in which there is an increased number of cells and glandular structures in the uterine lining. Endometrial hyperplasia can have either normal or atypical cells and simple or complex glandular structures. The risk for developing cancer in the lining of the uterus is higher when endometrial hyperplasia has atypical cells and complex glands.

There are 2 major types of uterine cancer:

- Adenocarcinoma. This type makes up more than 80% of uterine cancers. It develops from cells in the endometrium. This cancer is commonly called endometrial cancer. One common endometrial adenocarcinoma is called endometrioid carcinoma, and treatment varies depending on the grade of the tumor, how far it goes into the uterus, and the stage or extent of disease. Less common types of uterine cancers include serous, clear cell, and carcinosarcoma.
- Sarcoma. This type of uterine cancer develops in the supporting tissues of the uterine glands or in the myometrium, which is the uterine muscle. Sarcoma accounts for about 2% to 4% of uterine cancers. In most situations, sarcomas are treated differently from adenocarcinomas. Types of endometrial sarcoma include leiomyosarcoma, endometrial stromal sarcoma, and undifferentiated sarcoma. Learn more about sarcoma.

Cancer confined to the uterine cervix is treated differently from uterine cancer;

Symptoms Of Cancer

When cancer begins, it produces no symptoms. Signs and symptoms appear as the mass grows or ulcerates. The findings that result depend on the cancer's type and location. Few symptoms are specific. Many frequently occur in individuals who have other conditions. Cancer is a "great imitator". Thus, it is common for people diagnosed with cancer to have been treated for other diseases, which were hypothesized to be causing their symptoms.

People may become anxious or depressed post-diagnosis. The risk of suicide in people with cancer is approximately double.

Local symptoms

Local symptoms may occur due to the mass of the tumor or its ulceration. For example, mass effects from lung cancer can block the bronchus resulting in cough or pneumonia; esophageal cancer can cause narrowing of the esophagus, making it difficult or painful to swallow; and colorectal cancer may lead to narrowing or blockages in the bowel, affecting bowel habits. Masses in breasts or testicles may produce observable lumps. Ulceration can cause bleeding that, if it occurs in the lung, will lead to coughing up blood, in the bowels to anemia or rectal bleeding, in the bladder to blood in the urine and in the uterus to vaginal bleeding. Although localized pain may occur in advanced cancer, the initial swelling is usually painless. Some cancers can cause a buildup of fluid within the chest or abdomen.

Systemic symptoms

General symptoms occur due to effects that are not related to direct or metastatic spread. These may include: unintentional weight loss, fever, excessive fatigue and changes to the skin. Hodgkin disease, leukemias and cancers of the liver or kidney can cause a persistent fever.

Some cancers may cause specific groups of systemic symptoms, termed paraneoplastic syndrome. Examples include the appearance of myasthenia gravis in thymoma and clubbing in lung cancer.

Metastasis

Cancer can spread from its original site by local spread, lymphatic spread to regional lymph nodes or by hematogenous spread via the blood to distant sites, known as metastasis. When cancer spreads by a hematogenous route, it usually spreads all over the body. However, cancer 'seeds' grow in certain selected site only ('soil') as hypothesized in the soil and seed hypothesis of cancer metastasis. The symptoms of metastatic cancers depend on the tumor location and can include enlarged lymph nodes (which can be felt or sometimes seen under the skin and are typically hard), enlarged liver or enlarged spleen, which can be felt in the abdomen, pain or fracture of affected bones and neurological symptoms.

Causes Of Cancer

The majority of cancers, some 90–95% of cases, are due to genetic mutations from environmental and lifestyle factors. The remaining 5–10% are due to inherited genetics. Environmental, as used by cancer researchers, means any cause that is not inherited genetically, such as lifestyle, economic, and behavioral factors and not merely pollution. Common environmental factors that contribute to cancer death include tobacco (25–30%), diet and obesity (30–35%), infections (15–20%), radiation (both ionizing and non-ionizing, up to 10%), lack of physical activity, and pollution. Psychological stress does not appear to be a risk factor for the onset of cancer, though it may worsen outcomes in those who already have cancer.

It is not generally possible to prove what caused a particular cancer because the various causes do not have specific fingerprints. For example, if a person who uses tobacco heavily develops lung cancer, then it was probably caused by the tobacco use, but since everyone has a small chance of developing lung cancer as a result of air pollution or radiation, the cancer may have developed for one of those reasons. Excepting the rare transmissions that occur with pregnancies and occasional organ donors, cancer is generally not a transmissible disease.

Chemicals
Alcohol and cancer and Smoking and cancer

The incidence of lung cancer is highly correlated with smoking.

Exposure to particular substances have been linked to specific types of cancer. These substances are called carcinogens.

Tobacco smoke, for example, causes 90% of lung cancer. It also causes cancer in the larynx, head, neck, stomach, bladder, kidney, esophagus and pancreas. Tobacco smoke contains over fifty known carcinogens, including nitrosamines and polycyclic aromatic hydrocarbons.

Tobacco is responsible for about one in five cancer deaths worldwide and about one in three in the developed world. Lung cancer death rates in the United States have mirrored smoking patterns, with increases in smoking followed by dramatic increases in lung cancer death rates and, more recently, decreases in smoking rates since the 1950s followed by decreases in lung cancer death rates in men since 1990.

In Western Europe, 10% of cancers in males and 3% of cancers in females are attributed to alcohol exposure, especially liver and digestive tract cancers. Cancer from work-related substance exposures may cause between 2 and 20% of cases, causing at least 200,000 deaths. Cancers such as lung cancer and mesothelioma can come from inhaling tobacco smoke or asbestos fibers, or leukemia from exposure to benzene.

Diet and exercise

Diet, physical inactivity and obesity are related to up to 30–35% of cancer deaths. In the United States, excess body weight is associated with the development of many types of cancer and is a factor in 14–20% of cancer deaths. A UK study including data on over 5 million people showed higher body mass index to be related to at least 10 types of cancer and responsible for around

12,000 cases each year in that country. Physical inactivity is believed to contribute to cancer risk, not only through its effect on body weight but also through negative effects on the immune system and endocrine system. More than half of the effect from diet is due to overnutrition (eating too much), rather than from eating too few vegetables or other healthful foods.

Some specific foods are linked to specific cancers. A high-salt diet is linked to gastric cancer. Aflatoxin B1, a frequent food contaminant, causes liver cancer. Betel nut chewing can cause oral cancer. National differences in dietary practices may partly explain differences in cancer incidence. For example, gastric cancer is more common in Japan due to its high-salt diet while colon cancer is more common in the United States. Immigrant cancer profiles mirror those of their new country, often within one generation.

Infection

Worldwide approximately 18% of cancer deaths are related to infectious diseases. This proportion ranges from a high of 25% in Africa to less than 10% in the developed world. Viruses are the usual infectious agents that cause cancer but cancer bacteria and parasites may also play a role.

Oncoviruses (viruses that can cause cancer) include human papillomavirus (cervical cancer), Epstein–Barr virus (B-cell lymphoproliferative disease and nasopharyngeal carcinoma), Kaposi's sarcoma herpesvirus (Kaposi's sarcoma and primary effusion lymphomas), hepatitis B and hepatitis C viruses (hepatocellular carcinoma) and human T-cell leukemia virus-1 (T-cell leukemias). Bacterial infection may also increase the risk of cancer, as seen in Helicobacter pylori-induced gastric carcinoma.[50][51] Parasitic infections associated with cancer include Schistosoma haematobium (squamous cell carcinoma of the bladder) and the liver flukes, Opisthorchis viverrini and Clonorchis sinensis (cholangiocarcinoma).[52]

Radiation
Radiation-induced cancer

Radiation exposure such as ultraviolet radiation and radioactive material is a risk factor for cancer. Many non-melanoma skin cancers are due to ultraviolet radiation, mostly from sunlight. Sources of ionizing radiation include medical imaging and radon gas.

Ionizing radiation is not a particularly strong mutagen.Residential exposure to radon gas, for example, has similar cancer risks as passive smoking. Radiation is a more potent source of cancer when combined with other cancer-causing agents, such as radon plus tobacco smoke. Radiation can cause cancer in most parts of the body, in all animals and at any age. Children are twice as likely to develop radiation-induced leukemia as adults; radiation exposure before birth has ten times the effect.

Medical use of ionizing radiation is a small but growing source of radiation-induced cancers. Ionizing radiation may be used to treat other cancers, but this may, in some cases, induce a second form of cancer. It is also used in some kinds of medical imaging.

Prolonged exposure to ultraviolet radiation from the sun can lead to melanoma and other skin malignancies. Clear evidence establishes ultraviolet radiation, especially the non-ionizing medium wave UVB, as the cause of most non-melanoma skin cancers, which are the most common forms of cancer in the world.

Non-ionizing radio frequency radiation from mobile phones, electric power transmission and other similar sources has been described as a possible carcinogen by the World Health Organization's International Agency for Research on Cancer.Evidence, however, has not supported a concern. This includes that studies have not found a consistent link between mobile phone radiation and cancer risk.

Heredity

The vast majority of cancers are non-hereditary (sporadic). Hereditary cancers are primarily caused by an inherited genetic defect. Less than 0.3% of the population are carriers of a genetic mutation that has a large effect on cancer risk and these cause less than 3–10% of cancer. Some of these syndromes include: certain inherited mutations in the genes BRCA1 and BRCA2 with a more than 75% risk of breast cancer and ovarian cancer, and hereditary nonpolyposis colorectal cancer (HNPCC or Lynch syndrome), which is present in about 3% of people with colorectal cancer, among others.

Statistically for cancers causing most mortality, the relative risk of developing colorectal cancer when a first-degree relative (parent, sibling or child) has been diagnosed with it is about 2. The corresponding relative risk is 1.5 for lung cancer,[65] and 1.9 for prostate cancer.[66] For breast cancer, the relative risk is 1.8 with a first-degree relative having developed it at 50 years of age or older, and 3.3 when the relative developed it when being younger than 50 years of age.

Taller people have an increased risk of cancer because they have more cells than shorter people. Since height is genetically determined to a large extent, taller people have a heritable increase of cancer risk.

Physical Agents

Some substances cause cancer primarily through their physical, rather than chemical, effects. A prominent example of this is prolonged exposure to asbestos, naturally occurring mineral fibers that are a major cause of mesothelioma (cancer of the serous membrane) usually the serous membrane surrounding the lungs. Other substances in this category, including both naturally occurring and synthetic asbestos-like fibers, such as wollastonite, attapulgite, glass wool and rock wool, are believed to have similar effects. Non-fibrous particulate materials that cause cancer include powdered metallic cobalt and nickel and crystalline silica (quartz, cristobalite and tridymite). Usually, physical carcinogens must get inside the body (such as through inhalation) and require years of exposure to produce cancer.

Physical trauma resulting in cancer is relatively rare. Claims that breaking bones resulted in bone cancer, for example, have not been proven. Similarly, physical trauma is not accepted as a cause for cervical cancer, breast cancer or brain cancer. One accepted source is frequent, long-term application of hot objects to the body. It is possible that repeated burns on the same part of the body, such as those produced by kanger and kairo heaters (charcoal hand warmers), may produce skin cancer, especially if carcinogenic chemicals are also present. Frequent consumption of scalding hot tea may produce esophageal cancer. Generally, it is believed that cancer arises, or a pre-existing cancer is encouraged, during the process of healing, rather than directly by the trauma. However, repeated injuries to the same tissues might promote excessive cell proliferation, which could then increase the odds of a cancerous mutation.

Chronic inflammation has been hypothesized to directly cause mutation. Inflammation can contribute to proliferation, survival, angiogenesis and migration of cancer cells by influencing the tumor microenvironment. Oncogenes build up an inflammatory pro-tumorigenic microenvironment.

Hormones

Some hormones play a role in the development of cancer by promoting cell proliferation. Insulin-like growth factors and their binding proteins play a key role in cancer cell proliferation, differentiation and apoptosis, suggesting possible involvement in carcinogenesis.

Hormones are important agents in sex-related cancers, such as cancer of the breast, endometrium, prostate, ovary and testis and also of thyroid cancer and bone cancer. For example, the daughters of women who have breast cancer have significantly higher levels of estrogen and progesterone than the daughters of women without breast cancer. These higher hormone levels may explain their higher risk of breast cancer, even in the absence of a breast-cancer gene. Similarly, men of African ancestry have significantly higher levels of testosterone than men of European ancestry and have a correspondingly higher level of prostate cancer. Men of Asian ancestry, with the lowest levels of testosterone-activating androstanediol glucuronide, have the lowest levels of prostate cancer.

Other factors are relevant: obese people have higher levels of some hormones associated with cancer and a higher rate of those cancers. Women who take hormone replacement therapy have a higher risk of developing cancers associated with those hormones. On the other hand, people who exercise far more than average have lower levels of these hormones and lower risk of cancer.

Osteosarcoma may be promoted by growth hormones. Some treatments and prevention approaches leverage this cause by artificially reducing hormone levels and thus discouraging hormone-sensitive cancers.

Autoimmune diseases

There is an association between celiac disease and an increased risk of all cancers. People with untreated celiac disease have a higher risk, but this risk decreases with time after diagnosis and strict treatment, probably due to the adoption of a gluten-free diet, which seems to have a protective role against development of malignancy in people with celiac disease. However, the delay in diagnosis and initiation of a gluten-free diet seems to increase the risk of malignancies. Rates of gastrointestinal cancers are increased in people with Crohn's disease and ulcerative colitis, due to chronic inflammation. Also, immunomodulators and biologic agents used to treat these diseases may promote developing extra-intestinal malignancies.

Diagnosis of Cancer

Most cancers are initially recognized either because of the appearance of signs or symptoms or through screening. Neither of these leads to a definitive diagnosis, which requires the examination of a tissue sample by a pathologist. People with suspected cancer are investigated with medical tests. These commonly include blood tests, X-rays, (contrast) CT scans and endoscopy.

The tissue diagnosis from the biopsy indicates the type of cell that is proliferating, its histological grade, genetic abnormalities and other features. Together, this information is useful to evaluate the prognosis and to choose the best treatment.

Cytogenetics and immunohistochemistry are other types of tissue tests. These tests provide information about molecular changes (such as mutations, fusion genes and numerical chromosome changes) and may thus also indicate the prognosis and best treatment.

BEETROOT

Beetroot has been gaining in popularity as a superfood. Recent studies claim that beets and beetroot juice can improve athletic performance, reduce blood pressure, and increase blood flow.

So much so that an increasing number of juices and drinks are now incorporating this nutritious food.

Beetroot comes from the same family as sugar beets. However, it is genetically and nutritionally different. Sugar beets are white, and manufacturers tend to use them for extracting sugar and sweetening processed foods. It is not possible to extract sugar from beetroot, which is mostly red or gold.

Nutrition

One cup of raw beets provides:

- 58.5 calories
- 13 g of carbohydrates, including 9.19 g of sugar and 3.81 g of fiber
- 2.19 g of protein

Beetroot can also add the following vitamins and minerals to a person's diet.

Nutrient	Percentage of an adult's daily requirement
Vitamin C	7.4%
Vitamin A	0.3% for males, and 0.39% for females
Folate	37%
Magnesium	7.83% for males, and 10.97% for females
Phosphorus	7.77%

Beets also contain small amounts of:

- calcium
- iron
- thiamine
- riboflavin
- vitamin B-6
- copper
- selenium

Green, leafy vegetables such as beet tops provide high levels of dietary nitrate. Cooked beet tops are a great source of iron, vitamin C, vitamin A, magnesium, potassium, and folate.

When choosing a beetroot, make sure that it is heavy for its size and does not have signs of surface damage. If a beet still has its green tops, they should look fresh and not wilted. These are also edible and have significant nutritional value.

Benefits

Beetroot provides a wide range of possible health benefits, such as reducing blood pressure, improving digestion, and lowering the risk of diabetes.

The sections below discuss these potential benefits in more detail.

Heart health and blood pressure

A study of 68 people with high blood pressure examined the effects of drinking 250 milliliters of beetroot juice every day.

The researchers found that doing so significantly lowered blood pressure after ingestion.

They suggest that this antihypertensive effect was due to the high levels of nitrate in the beet juice. They recommend consuming high nitrate vegetables as an effective, low cost way to help treat high blood pressure.

However, people should never stop taking a prescribed blood pressure medication without first talking to a doctor.

High blood pressure is a primary risk factor for cardiovascular disease (CVD). Reducing it by making dietary changes and through other means can help prevent heart failure, stroke, heart attacks, and other life threatening complications of CVD.

Diabetes

Beets contain an antioxidant called alpha-lipoic acid. This compound may help lower glucose levels and increase insulin sensitivity.

A review of studies looked at the effects of alpha-lipoic acid on the symptoms of diabetic neuropathy. The researchers found that oral and intravenous administration of alpha-lipoic acid supplements led to a decrease in symptoms of peripheral and autonomic neuropathy in people with diabetes.

However, most of the doses in these studies were far higher than those that are available in beetroot. The effects of smaller dietary doses are not yet clear from the available research.

Digestion and regularity

One cup of beetroot provides 3.81 grams (g) of fiber. Consuming enough fiber is essential for smooth digestion and gut health.

A single cup of beets can provide more than 8.81% of a person's daily requirement of fiber, depending on their age and sex.

Including beetroot in the diet is one way that a person can increase their fiber intake.

Exercise and athletic performance

Many studies have found that beetroot juice supplementation can improve the amount of oxygen that muscles absorb during exercise. A study found that high doses of beetroot juice improved the time trial results of experienced cyclists.

Cancer prevention

A 2019 review of studies found that certain compounds in beets can disrupt the cancerous mutations of cells. Such compounds include betalains, which are pigments that give beets their red and yellow color.

Health professionals recommend beets as a replacement for cancer risk reduction.

CARROT

The carrot (Daucus carota) is a root vegetable often claimed to be the perfect health food.

It is crunchy, tasty, and highly nutritious. Carrots are a particularly good source of beta carotene, fiber, vitamin K1, potassium, and antioxidants.

They also have a number of health benefits. They're a weight-loss-friendly food and have been linked to lower cholesterol levels and improved eye health.

What's more, their carotene antioxidants have been linked to a reduced risk of cancer.

Carrots are found in many colors, including yellow, white, orange, red, and purple.

Carrots get their bright color from beta carotene, an antioxidant that your body converts into vitamin A.

Nutrition

Carrots' water content ranges from 86–95%, and the edible portion consists of around 10% carbs.

Carrots contain very little fat and protein.

The nutrition facts for two small-to-medium raw carrots (100 grams) are:

- Calories: 41
- Water: 88%
- Protein: 0.9 grams
- Carbs: 9.6 grams
- Sugar: 4.7 grams
- Fiber: 2.8 grams
- Fat: 0.2 grams

Carbs

Carrots are mainly composed of water and carbs.

The carbs consist of starch and sugars, such as sucrose and glucose.

They are also a relatively good source of fiber, with one medium-sized carrot (61 grams) providing 2 grams.

Carrots often rank low on the glycemic index (GI), which is a measure of how quickly foods raise blood sugar after a meal.

Their GI ranges from 16–60 — lowest for raw carrots, a little higher for cooked ones, and highest for puréed.

Eating low-glycemic foods is linked to numerous health benefits and considered particularly beneficial for people with diabetes.

Fiber

Pectin is the main form of soluble fiber in carrots.

Soluble fibers can lower blood sugar levels by slowing down your digestion of sugar and starch.

They can also feed the friendly bacteria in your gut, which may lead to improved health and decreased risk of disease.

What's more, certain soluble fibers can impair the absorption of cholesterol from your digestive tract, lowering blood cholesterol.

The main insoluble fibers in carrots are cellulose, hemicellulose, and lignin. Insoluble fibers may reduce your risk of constipation and promote regular bowel movements.

Vitamins and Minerals

Carrots are a good source of several vitamins and minerals, especially biotin, potassium, and vitamins A (from beta carotene), K1 (phylloquinone), and B6.

- Vitamin A: Carrots are rich in beta carotene, which your body converts into vitamin A. This nutrient promotes good vision and is important for growth, development, and immune function.
- Biotin: A B vitamin formerly known as vitamin H, biotin plays an important role in fat and protein metabolism.
- Vitamin K1: Also known as phylloquinone, vitamin K1 is important for blood coagulation and can promote bone health.
- Potassium: An essential mineral, potassium is important for blood pressure control.
- Vitamin B6: A group of related vitamins, B6 is involved in the conversion of food into energy.

Other Plant Compounds

Carrots offer many plant compounds, including carotenoids.

These are substances with powerful antioxidant activity that have been linked to improved immune function and reduced risk of many illnesses, including heart disease, various degenerative ailments, and certain types of cancer.

Beta carotene, the main carotene in carrots, can be converted into vitamin A in your body.

However, this conversion process may vary by individual. Eating fat with carrots can help you absorb more of the beta carotene.

The main plant compounds in carrots are:

- Beta carotene: Orange carrots are very high in beta carotene. The absorption is better (up to 6.5-fold) if the carrots are cooked.
- Alpha-carotene: An antioxidant that, like beta carotene, is partly converted into vitamin A in your body.
- Lutein: One of the most common antioxidants in carrots, lutein is predominantly found in yellow and orange carrots and is important for eye health.
- Lycopene: A bright red antioxidant found in many red fruits and vegetables, including red and purple carrots,

lycopene may decrease your risk of cancer and heart disease.
- **Polyacetylenes:** Recent research has identified bioactive compounds in carrots that may help protect against leukemia and other cancers.
- **Anthocyanins:** These are powerful antioxidants found in dark-colored carrots.

Health benefits of carrots

Much of the research on carrots has focused on carotenoids.

Reduced risk of cancer

Diets rich in carotenoids may help protect against several types of cancer.

This includes prostate, colon, and stomach cancers.

Women with high circulating levels of carotenoids may also have a reduced risk of breast cancer.

Dated research suggested that carotenoids could protect against lung cancer, but newer studies have not identified a correlation.

Lower blood cholesterol

High blood cholesterol is a well-known risk factor for heart disease.

Intake of carrots has been linked to lower cholesterol levels.

Weight loss

As a low-calorie food, carrots can increase fullness and decrease calorie intake in subsequent meals.

For this reason, they may be a useful addition to an effective weight loss diet.

Eye health

Individuals with low vitamin A levels are more likely to experience night blindness, a condition that may diminish by eating carrots or other foods rich in vitamin A or carotenoids.

Carotenoids may also cut your risk of age-related macular degeneration.

APPLE

Apples are a popular fruit, containing antioxidants, vitamins, dietary fiber, and a range of other nutrients. Due to their varied nutrient content, they may help prevent several health conditions.

Apples come in a variety of shapes, colors, and flavors and provide a range of nutrients that can benefit many different aspects of a person's health.

For example, they may help reduce the risk of cancer, obesity, heart disease, diabetes, and several other conditions.

In this article, learn more about the nutritional content of apples and how they may benefit a person's health.

Nutrition

The table below shows the amount of each nutrient in a medium sized raw apple weighing around 182 g.

It also shows how much an adult needs of each nutrient, according to the 2015–2020 Dietary Guidelines for Americans. Needs vary according to the individual's age and sex.

Nutrient	Amount in 1 apple	Daily adult requirement
Energy (calories)	94.6	1,800–3,000
Carbohydrate (g)	25.1, including 18.9 g of sugar	130
Fiber (g)	4.4	22.4–33.6
Calcium (milligrams [mg])	10.9	1,000–1,300
Phosphorus (mg)	20	700
Magnesium (mg)	9.1	320–420
Potassium (mg)	195	4,700
Vitamin C (mg)	8.37	75–90
Folate (micrograms [mcg])	5.46	400
Choline	6.19	425–550

Beta-carotene (mcg)	49.1	No data
Lutein and zeaxanthin (mcg)	52.8	No data
Vitamin K (mcg)	4	90–120

Applies also provide iron, vitamin A, some B vitamins, and vitamin E.

Benefits

Apples are rich in fiber, vitamins, and minerals, all of which benefit health. They also provide an array of antioxidants. These substances help neutralize free radicals.

Free radicals are reactive molecules that can build up as a result of natural processes and environmental pressures. If too many free radicals accumulate in the body, they can cause oxidative stress, and this can lead to cell damage. This damage can contribute to a range of conditions, including cancer and diabetes.

Apples contain a range of antioxidants, including:

- quercetin

- catechin
- phloridzin
- chlorogenic acid

The sections below look at previous research into apples' potential health benefits.

Neurological health and dementia

A laboratory study concluded that quercetin has a neuroprotective effect, possibly because it prevents the creation of reactive species. It appears to help neurons survive and continue to function. It may therefore help prevent age-related neuron loss.

The results of a mouse study suggested that high dose quercetin supplementation may help protect cells from the type of damage that can lead to Alzheimer's disease.

It is worth noting that most studies of this type used high doses of quercetin that are unlikely to be present in normal dietary sources. In addition, scientists need to do more studies in humans before they can confirm that quercetin improves neurological health in people.

Stroke

An older study from 2000 looked at how consuming apples over 28 years affected the risk of stroke in 9,208 people.

Apples contain many nutrients that may lower the risk of stroke. One review found, for example, that people who consume the most fiber appear to have a lower risk of cardiovascular disease, coronary heart disease, and stroke.

A medium sized apple around 3 inches in diameter and weighing 182 grams (g) provides 4.37 g of fiber. That is around 13–20% of an adult's daily requirement, depending on their age and sex.

Cholesterol

One study found that eating raw apples lowered levels of low-density lipoprotein cholesterol among healthy people, but that drinking clear apple juice did not have the same impact. The authors therefore conclude that it is the fiber in apples that helps reduce cholesterol.

Heart health

Apples contain fiber, vitamin C, antioxidants, and potassium. A medium sized apple provides the following:

- 13–20% of a person's daily fiber needs
- 9–11% of a person's daily vitamin C needs
- 4% of a person's daily potassium needs

Fiber appears to help manage blood pressure, which may reduce the risk of cardiovascular disease.

Vitamin C is an antioxidant that, alongside other antioxidants, may play a role in protecting some aspects of heart health. Vitamin C may also boost the immune system and help defend the body from infections and diseases.

Potassium helps relax the blood vessels, reducing the risk of high blood pressure and cardiovascular complications.

Diabetes

In 2013, a population study found that people who replaced three servings per week of fruit juice with the same amount of whole fruit, including apples, had a 7% lower risk of developing type 2 diabetes than those who did not eat fruit.

Also, those who consume the most fiber have a lower risk of developing type 2 diabetes, suggested one 2011 review. People who already have diabetes and follow a high fiber diet may also have lower blood sugar levels.

A medium apple contains 25.1 g of carbohydrate, of which 18.9 g is sugar. However, it also provides fiber and other nutrients, which means that, as a sweet snack, it has additional health benefits.

Cancer

Consuming antioxidant-rich foods may help prevent the oxidative stress that causes cell damage and may lead to the development of certain cancers. Apples are a good source of antioxidants.

One meta-analysis from 2016 concluded that consuming apples may help lower the risk of lung cancer, breast cancer, and colorectal cancer, among other types.

Obesity

According to a rodent study, apples contain bioactive compounds that may help promote healthful gut bacteria, which may help optimize the health of people with obesity.

The researchers looked at how eating apples might affect the gut microbiota of rats. The changes they observed suggested that apple consumption may help humans with obesity.

Fiber can also help a person feel full for longer, making them less likely to overeat.

Dietary tips and recipes

There are many varieties of apples, as well as several different ways of consuming them.

People can eat them raw, as applesauce, chopped in salads, baked whole, in pies, pastries, and cakes, in curries and chutneys, dried in slices, added to smoothies, and as juice.

Some popular apple varieties include:

McIntosh: A juicy, red apple with tender, white flesh and a tangy flavor.

Red delicious: A crisp, juicy red apple.

Fuji: Yellow and red in color, it has firm, sweet flesh.

Granny Smith: A green apple with crisp, greenish flesh and a sharp flavor.

Golden delicious: A yellow apple with a mild, sweet flavor.

Preferences vary, but many people prefer tart, tangy apples for making applesauce or apple pie. To avoid adding sugar, try pairing tart apples with sweet ones in cooking or adding spices to counter the sharpness.

LEMON

Lemons are a popular fruit that people use in small quantities to add flavor to food. However, they rarely consume them alone due to their intense, sour taste.

Lemons give flavor to baked goods, sauces, salad dressings, marinades, drinks, and desserts, and they are also a good source of vitamin C.

One 58 gram (g) lemon can provide over 30 milligrams (mg) of vitamin C.

Vitamin C is essential for health, and a deficiency can lead to health problems. The early explorers knew this and took lemons on their long voyages to help prevent or treat scurvy, a life threatening condition that was common among sailors.

Nutrition

One lemon weighing 58 grams (g) contains:

- energy: 16.8 calories (kcal)
- carbohydrates: 5.41 g, of which 1.45 g are sugars
- calcium 15.1 milligrams (mg)
- iron: 0.35 mg

- magnesium: 4.6 mg
- phosphorus: 9.3 mg
- potassium: 80 mg
- selenium: 0.2 micrograms (mcg)
- vitamin C: 30.7 mg
- folate: 6.4 mcg
- choline: 3.0 mg
- vitamin A: 0.6 mcg
- lutein + zeaxanthin: 6.4 mcg

Current dietary guidelines recommend an intake of 75 mg of vitamin C per day for women aged 19 years and older and 90 mg per day for men.

Smokers need 35 mg per day more than nonsmokers.

Lemons also contain small amounts of thiamin, riboflavin, vitamin B-6, pantothenic acid, copper, and manganese.

Benefits

Lemons are an excellent source of vitamin C and flavonoids, which are antioxidants.

Antioxidants help remove free radicals that can damage cells from the body.

These nutrients can help prevent diseases and boost health and wellbeing.

Here some of the possible benefits of consuming lemons.

Lowering stroke risk

According to a study, the flavonoids in citrus fruits may help lower the risk of ischemic stroke in women.

A study of data from nearly 70,000 women over 14 years showed that those who ate the most citrus fruits had a 19% lower risk of ischemic stroke than women who consumed the least.

Ischemic stroke is the most common type of stroke. It can happen when a blood clot blocks the flow of blood to the brain.

A population study showed that long term, regular consumption of foods that contain flavonoids might help protect against cancer and cardiovascular disease. However, the study indicated that people who smoked or consumed a lot of alcohol were less likely to benefit.

Blood pressure

One study found that women in Japan who walked regularly and consumed lemon every day had lower blood pressure than those who did not.

Cancer prevention

Lemons and lemon juice are an excellent source of the antioxidant vitamin C.

Antioxidants may help prevent free radicals from causing cell damage that can lead to cancer. However, exactly how antioxidants can help prevent cancer remains unclear.

Maintaining a healthy complexion

Vitamin C plays a vital role in the formation of collagen, the support system of the skin.

Sun exposure, pollution, age, and other factors can result in skin damage. A mouse study suggested that either eating vitamin C in its natural form or applying it topically can help prevent this type of damage.

Preventing asthma

People with asthma who consume higher amounts of vitamin C and other nutrients when they have a cold may experience fewer asthma attacks, according to a review.

The researchers found evidence that vitamin C also benefitted people with bronchial hypersensitivity when they also had a common cold.

Increasing iron absorption

Iron deficiency is a leading cause of anemia.

Pairing foods that are high in vitamin C with iron-rich foods maximizes the body's ability to absorb iron.

However, a high intake of vitamin C can trigger gastrointestinal problems in people who are taking iron supplements. For this reason, it is best to obtain iron from dietary sources, such as beef liver, lentils, raisins, dried beans, animal meats, and spinach.

Squeezing a little lemon juice onto a salad containing baby spinach leaves can help maximize the intake of both iron and vitamin C.

Boosting the immune system

Foods that are high in vitamin C and other antioxidants may help strengthen the immune system against the germs that cause the common cold and the flu.

A review found that, while vitamin C supplements do not appear the reduce the incidence of colds in a population, they may help reduce the length of time a cold lasts. Vitamin C may also help boost immunity in people who are undergoing extreme physical activity.

Squeezing a whole lemon into a glass of hot water with a large spoonful of honey makes a soothing drink for someone with a cough or cold.

Weight loss

In a study, rodents who consumed lemon peel phenols with a high fat diet for 12 weeks gained less weight than those who did not consume lemon.

In 2016, 84 premenopausal Korean women with a high body mass index (BMI) followed a lemon detox diet or another diet for 7 days. Those who followed the lemon detox diet experienced greater improvements in insulin resistance, body fat, BMI, body weight, and waist-hip ratio than those on the other diets.

Vitamin C

Vitamin C is an essential nutrient and an antioxidant.

Scurvy

If a person does not consume enough vitamin C, they will develop a deficiency, which is known as scurvy. It is rare in the United States, but it can affect people who do not have a varied diet.

Symptoms can start to appear within a month of not consuming vitamin C, and they include:

- fatigue
- malaise (a feeling of being unwell)
- inflammation of the gums or bleeding gums
- red patches on the skin due to blood vessels breaking beneath the surface
- joint pain
- slow wound healing
- loosening of teeth
- depression

Many of these happen when the connective tissues weaken due to the lack of vitamin C.

Since vitamin C helps the body absorb iron, people who are deficient in iron may also develop anemia.

BEETROOT, CARROT, APPLE AND LEMON FOR CANCER

Cancer is a disease that results in an uncontrollable growth of cells. There isn't any real proof of the Miracle Drink being able to cure cancer. However, it has been able to slow down the growth of cancerous cells. There was a case of a patient recovering from lung cancer after being instructed by a Chinese herbalist to drink the miracle juice. But the effectiveness of this precious elixir depends on the stage of cancer you are at.

This potion restores lost hope for people suffering from cancer. Not only proven applicable in the treatment of lung cancer, but also prevents the development of almost all kinds of malignant tumor cells. Beet comprising amino acid betaine having anticancer properties. Beetroot is a traditional cure for leukemia.

So, combining the three to harness all these benefits in one go, sounds like a good idea. Claims supported by recent research are followed by the delicious recipe to easily prepare the miracle drink at home in just five minutes.

However, we have also did stumble upon case of a Chinese herbalist recommending miracle drink to a patient of Lung cancer. And surprisingly, he recovered from the lethal disease in three months. Although, the extent of influence depends considerably on the stage of carcinoma and organ affected, but a real proof of such kind does call for a toast of miracle drink everyday.

How Does The Miracle Drink Fight Cancer?

The main ingredient of this juice that fights cancer is beetroot. In fact, this vegetable has been used a cancer treatment for centuries in Europe. Research has found that beets contain a flavonoid known as betazyane that inhibits the growth of tumors and increases the intake of oxygen within the cells. This, in turn, protects the levels of Vitamin C, which is another nutrient that effectively fights cancer.

Beetroot juice is also rich in iron. This helps in the regeneration of red blood corpuscles that supply more oxygen to cancer cells. When the oxygen content is increased, it helps in improving cellular respiration, which in turn helps in destroying cancer cells.

How To Make Miracle Drink For Cancer

Making ABC is as simple as its name! All you need is apples, beetroots, and carrots.

1. First, make sure that the three ingredients are thoroughly washed and cleaned.

2. Slice them into small pieces. Do not peel them as a majority of the goodness of these foods is contained in their peels.

3. Blend them in a juicer and add a small amount of water to improve its consistency, making it easier to drink.

4. If you like, you can add a tablespoon of honey or fresh lemon juice to improve its taste.

Recipe of ABC Miracle Drink

Ingredients you'll need:

1. Red Apple (1 medium size)

2. Beet Root (1 medium size)

3. Carrot (1 medium size)

4. Lemon juice or Honey for taste (1 tbsp)

How to Prepare:

1. Wash the skin of vegetables and slice them in small pieces.
2. Blend them in juice grinder and add water to reduce consistency.
3. Take that juice in a glass and add honey or lemon juice
4. Enjoy the Miracle ABC juice!

When to Drink it:

Drink it on empty stomach in the morning. After one hour, you can have your breakfast. There is absolutely no side effect. Highly nutritious and easily absorbed. Very effective if you need to loose weight. It will boost your immune system after a 2 week routine.

Note: Please make sure to drink immediately from the juicer for best effect.

Dosage

The infusion of beetroot, carrot, apple and lemon drink in the morning, on an empty stomach. Have breakfast after an hour. The beverage can be drink twice a day. The second time you drink at 17 pm.

It is recommended to drink it slowly and every sip briefly retain in the mouth.

Treatment with juice should continuously take from one to three months, if you want to achieve long-term beneficial effects on your health.

CONCLUSION

It's recommended for people with lung cancer, as well as all the other Cancer patients that are going through the harsh treatment.

In all types of cancer, some of the body's cells begin to divide without stopping and spread into surrounding tissues.

It makes your immune system much stronger if you drink it a glass of this Miracle drink for 3 months, religiously each morning as soon as you wake up and before you eat or drink anything.

It will also help patients cope with the side effects of cancer treatment.

CPSIA information can be obtained
at www.ICGtesting.com
Printed in the USA
BVHW041744210523
664595BV00004B/125